Air Fryer Cookbook for Beginners 2021

Enjoy the Crispness of Easy and Mouth-watering Recipes. Burn Fat without Feeling Hungry, Regain Confidence and Lose Weight Fast

Jessica Harris

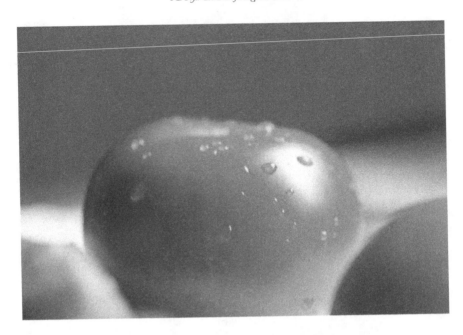

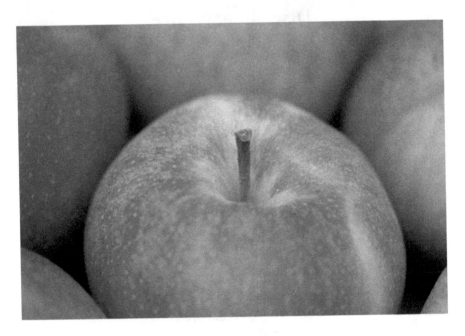

Table of Contents

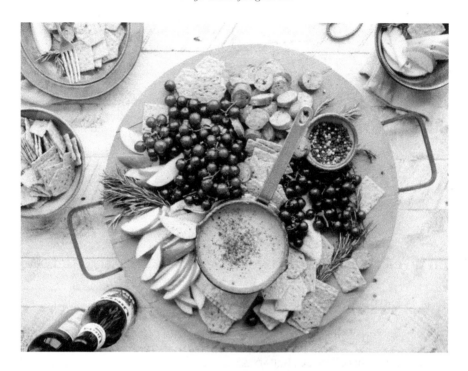

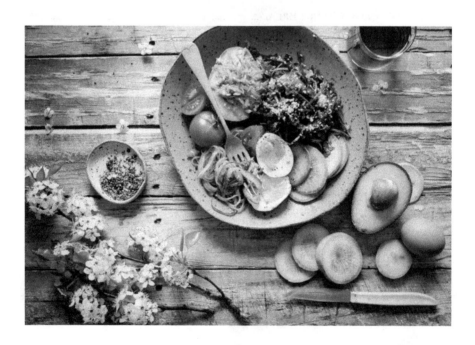

Introduction

The multi-functional Instant Vortex Air Fryer is made to start your adventure in cooking. To do so successfully, though, you must start learning all the functions and options that this great kitchen helper has. Yes, it is exciting, and we all want to rush off and start cooking and baking, which is excellent. Staring at the results of flopped recipes is not so great, though. See what you may need to buy extra and take to heart the tips from people who learned the hard way to do and what not to do.

The Vortex comes pre-programmed with ten smart programs for each of the different cooking modes. This includes default temperatures and cooking times for each of the cooking modes. This makes it very easy to use this multi-functional appliance as it takes the guesswork out of which cooking mode to use and what the optimal temperature for any specific cooking mode is.

The programming also tells you when to place the food inside the Vortex air fryer oven, when to turn food over or rotate the cooking trays, and when to remove the food from the air fryer oven.

There is currently no other appliance on the market that incorporates seven different cooking modes in one appliance. You would need several various appliances for the same functions that the Vortex offers.

You do not have to go out to get fast food; you can make a healthier option at home. The rotisserie presents you with a crisp whole chicken and roast meat without a stove oven. You can switch instantly between cooking different types of food; there is no need to invest in several appliances.

The Vortex cooks faster, so you can have deep-fried tasting food much quicker than conventional deep-frying.

Cleaning the Vortex is not a major chore. There is no scrubbing with harsh chemicals, and all the accessories are dishwasher safe. Cleaning by hand is just as quick with a cloth and soapy water.

Chapter 1. Breakfast and Brunch

1. Pork Meatballs

Basic Recipe

Preparation Time: 10 minutes

Cooking Time: 20 minutes

Servings: 4

Ingredients:

- 12 ounces ground pork

- 1/2 cup Panko bread crumbs

- 1 Egg

- 1 teaspoon salt

- 1 teaspoon dried parsley

- 1/2 teaspoon paprika

Directions:

1. Preheat the air fryer oven to 175 ° C. Mix ground pork, panko breadcrumbs, eggs, salt, parsley, and paprika in a large bowl and mix well.

2. Make 12 large meatballs with a scoop of ice cream.

3. Place the meatballs on a baking sheet, place half of the meatballs in the basket, and cook for 8 minutes

4. Shake the basket and cook for another 2 minutes Place on a serving plate and let rest for 5 minutes. Repeat with the remaining meatballs.

Nutrition:

Calories 64

Fat 1.6g

Carbs 3.3g

Protein 8.5g

2. Raspberry Smoked Pork Chops

Basic Recipe

Preparation Time: 15 minutes

Cooking Time: 15 minutes

Servings: 4

Ingredients:

- Cooking spray

- 2 large eggs

- 1/4 cup Coconut milk

- 1 cup Panko bread crumbs

- 1 cup finely chopped walnuts

- 4 Smoked bone-in pork chops (7-1/2 ounces each)

- 1/4 cup Coconut flour

- 2 tablespoons Stevia

- 2 tablespoons Raspberry

- 1 tablespoon Fresh orange juice

Directions:

1. Preheat the fryer to 400 °. Spray some oil in the frying basket.

2. Mix the eggs and coconut milk in a flat bowl. Mix the panko breadcrumbs with walnuts in another flat bowl and cover the pork chops with the flour. Shake off excess.

3. Dip into the egg mixture and then into the crumb mixture and tap on it to help it stick. If necessary,

4. Work in batches and place the chops in a single layer in the basket of the air fryer oven. Spray with oil, cook for 12 to 15 minutes until golden brown, turn after half the cooking time and sprinkle with additional cooking spray.

5. Remove and keep warm.

6. Repeat with the remaining chops. In the meantime, put the remaining ingredients in a small saucepan. Bring to a boil. Boil and stir until it gets a little thick, 6-8 minutes. Serve with chops.

Nutrition:

Calories 542

Fat 31.8g

Carbs 24.9g

Protein 41.3g

3. Crispy Pork Chops

Basic Recipe

Preparation Time: 15 minutes **Cooking Time:** 10 minutes

Servings: 4

Ingredients:

- 1 1/2 lb. Boneless pork chops

- 1/3 cup Almond Flour

- 1/4 cup Grated Parmesan cheese

- 1 teaspoon Garlic powder

- 1 teaspoon Paprika

Directions:

1. Preheat your air fryer to 350 degrees F.

2. In the meantime, mix all the ingredients, excluding pork chops in a large airtight bag. Place the pork chops in the bag, close them, and shake to cover the pork chops. Discard from the bag and put in one layer in the air fryer. Cook at least 12 minutes, according to the density of your pork chops.

Nutrition: Calories 204 Fat 7.4g Carbs 1.9g Protein 31.5g

4. Chicken Fried Rice

Basic Recipe

Preparation Time: 15 minutes

Cooking Time: 12 minutes

Servings: 4

Ingredients:

- 3 cups Cooked brown rice cold

- 1 cup cooked chicken diced

- 1 cup Cauliflower and carrots

- 6 tablespoons low sodium soy sauce

- 1 tablespoon Avocado oil

- 1/2 cup Onion diced

Directions:

1. Put the cooked brown rice in the bowl, add the avocado oil and soy sauce and mix well.

2. Put the peas & carrots, the diced onion and the diced chicken and mix greatly.

3. Put the rice mixture into the non-stick pan

4. Place the pan in the air fryer.

5. Set the fryer to 360 f with a cooking time of 20 minutes. When the timer is off, remove the pan from the fryer. Serve and enjoy!

Nutrition:

Calories 147

Fat 1.3g

Carbs 9.1g

Protein 10.1g

5. Steak and Asparagus Bundles

Basic Recipe

Preparation Time: 15 minutes

Cooking Time: 15 minutes

Servings: 4

Ingredients:

- 2 - 2 1/2 pounds Flank steak - cut into 6 pieces
- Kosher salt/black pepper
- 2 cloves Garlic - crushed
- 1-pound Asparagus - trimmed
- 3 Bell peppers - seeded and sliced thinly
- 1/3 cup Beef broth
- 2 tablespoons unsalted butter
- Olive oil spray

Directions:

1. Season the fillets with salt and pepper and place in a large zippered bag.

2. Add garlic. Close the bag and massage the fillets so that they are completely covered.

3. Put in the fridge and marinate for at least 1 hour overnight. When you're done, remove the marinade fillets and place them on a chopping board or sheet.

4. Throw away the marinade. Spread the mass evenly and place the asparagus and peppers in the middle of each steak.

5. Roll the steak around the vegetables and secure them.

6. Preheat the fryer. Depending on the size of your air fryer, the packages are stacked in the frying basket.

7. Spray the vegetables with olive oil. Cook for 5 minutes at 400 degrees.

8. Remove the meat packaging and let it rest for 5 minutes before serving/cutting. Heat in a small to medium-hot pan: balsamic vinegar, broth, and butter over medium heat.

9. Mix and continue cooking until the sauce thicken and halves. Season it with salt and pepper and pour the sauce over the meat packets before serving.

Nutrition:

Calories 220

Fat 10g

Carbs 3.8g Protein 27.6g

6. Pork Loin

Basic Recipe

Preparation Time: 5 minutes

Cooking Time: 20 minutes

Servings: 4

Ingredients:

- 1.5 lb. Pork tenderloin,

- Cooking spray

- 2 Small heads roasted garlic

- Salt & pepper

Directions:

1. Pat the Pork loin dry.

2. Cover all sides lightly with a non-stick coating, salt, and pepper on both sides.

3. Brushing with roasted garlic

4. Spray the rack and place it in.

5. Bake on vortex air fry press, at 350°F for at least 10 minutes for each side. Safely take off from the air fryer.

6. Remove carefully from the air fryer. Coming back to the fryer and Bake it for another 10 minutes

Nutrition:

Calories 220

Fat 10g

Carbs 3.9g

Protein 27.6g

7. Lemon-Garlic Chicken Thighs

Basic Recipe

Preparation Time: 10 minutes

Cooking Time: 25 minutes

Servings: 4

Ingredients:

- ¼ cup Lemon juice

- 2 tablespoons Coconut oil

- 1 teaspoon Dijon mustard

- 2 cloves Garlic, minced

- ¼ teaspoon Salt

- ⅛ Teaspoon Ground black pepper

- 4 Skin-on, bone-in chicken thighs

- 4 Lime wedges

Directions:

1. Put lemon juice, coconut oil, Dijon mustard, garlic, salt, and pepper in a container and mix well.

2. Reserve the marinade and put the chicken legs in a large plastic bag with a zipper. Put the marinade over the chicken and close the bag. Make sure all chicken bits are covered. Put in the freeze for at most 120 min.

3. Preheat an air fryer oven to 175 ° C.

4. Take the chicken out of the marinade and rub dry with a kitchen towel. Put the chicken bits in the frying basket and cook as needed.

5. Roast for 22 to 24 minutes until the chicken in the bone is cooked, and the juice is clear.

6. Press a lime wedge on each slice before serving.

Nutrition:

Calories 222

Fat 16.8g

Carbs 1.5g

Protein 15.9g

8. Steak and Mushrooms

Basic Recipe

Preparation Time: 5 minutes

Cooking Time: 10 minutes

Servings: 4

Ingredients:

- 1-pound beef sirloin steak, cut into 1-inch cubes

- 8 ounces Button mushrooms, sliced

- 1/4 cup Worcestershire sauce

- 1 tablespoon Olive oil

- 1 teaspoon Parsley flakes

- 1 teaspoon Paprika

- 1 teaspoon Crushed Chile flakes

Directions:

1. Mix steak, mushrooms, Worcestershire sauce, coconut oil, parsley, paprika, and chili flakes in a big bowl.

2. Cover and freeze for at least 4 hours or overnight. Remove from fridge 30 minutes before cooking.

3. Preheat the air fryer to 200 ° C. Dry out the marinade of the meat mixture and throw away. Place the steak and mushrooms in the frying basket and cook in the preheated air fryer for 5 minutes

4. Mix and cook for another 5 minutes. Place the steak and mushrooms on a plate and let them rest for 5 minutes

Nutrition:

Calories 269

Fat 10.8g

Carbs 5.2g

Protein 36.3g

9. Crispy Salt and Pepper Tofu

Basic Recipe

Preparation Time: 5 minutes

Cooking Time: 20 minutes

Servings: 4

Ingredients:

- ¼ cup chickpea flour

- ¼ cup arrowroot (or cornstarch)

- 1 teaspoon sea salt

- 1 teaspoon granulated garlic

- ½ teaspoon freshly grated black pepper

- 1 (15-ounce) package tofu, firm or extra-firm

- Cooking oil spray (sunflower, safflower, or refined coconut)

- Asian Spicy Sweet Sauce, optional

Directions:

1. In a medium bowl, combine the flour, arrowroot, salt, garlic, and pepper. Stir well to combine. Cut the tofu into cubes (no need to press—if it's a bit watery, that's fine!). Place the cubes into the flour mixture. Toss well to coat. Spray the tofu with

oil and toss again. (The spray will help the coating better stick to the tofu.)

2. Spray the air fryer basket with the oil. Place the tofu in a single layer in the air fryer basket (you may have to do this in 2 batches, depending on the size of your appliance) and spray the tops with oil. Fry for 8 minutes. Remove the air fryer basket and spray again with oil. Toss gently or turn the pieces over. Spray with oil again and fry for another 7 minutes, or until golden-browned and very crisp. Serve immediately, either plain or with the Asian Spicy Sweet Sauce.

Nutrition:

Calories 148

Fat 5g

Carbs 14g

Protein 11g

10. Bacon 'n Egg-Substitute Bake

Basic Recipe

Preparation Time: 5 minutes

Cooking Time: 30 minutes

Servings: 4

Ingredients:

- 1 (6 ounce) package Canadian bacon, quartered

- 1/2 cup 2% milk

- 1/4 teaspoon ground mustard

- 1/4 teaspoon salt

- 2 cups shredded Cheddar-Monterey Jack cheese blend

- 3/4 cup and 2 tablespoons egg substitute (such as Egg Beaters® Southwestern Style)

- 4 frozen hash brown patties

Directions:

1. Lightly grease the baking pan of the air fryer with cooking spray.

2. Evenly spread hash brown patties on the bottom of the pan. Top evenly with bacon and then followed by cheese.

3. In a bowl, whisk well mustard, salt, milk, and egg substitute. Pour over bacon mixture.

4. Cover air fryer baking pan with foil.

5. Preheat air fryer to 330F.

6. Cook for another 20 minutes, remove foil and continue cooking for another 15 minutes or until eggs are set.

7. Serve and enjoy.

Nutrition:

Calories 459

Carbs 21.0g

Protein 29.4g

Fat 28.5g

11. Buttered Spinach-Egg Omelet

Basic Recipe

Preparation Time: 5 minutes **Cooking Time:** 10 minutes

Servings: 4

Ingredients:

- ¼ cup coconut milk

- 1 tablespoon melted butter

- 1-pound baby spinach, chopped finely

- 3 tablespoons olive oil

- 4 eggs, beaten

- Salt and pepper to taste

Directions:

1. Preheat the air fryer for 5 minutes. In a mixing bowl, combine the eggs, coconut milk, olive oil, and butter until well-combined. Add the spinach and season with salt and pepper to taste. Pour all ingredients into a baking dish that will fit in the air fryer. Bake at 350F for 15 minutes.

Nutrition: Calories 310 Carbs 3.6g Protein 13.6g Fat 26.8g

12. Cheeseburger Egg Rolls

Basic Recipe

Preparation Time: 10 minutes

Cooking Time: 7 minutes

Servings: 6

Ingredients:

- 6 egg roll wrappers

- 6 chopped dill pickle chips

- 1 tbsp. yellow mustard

- 3 tbsp. cream cheese

- 3 tbsp. shredded cheddar cheese

- ½ C. chopped onion

- ½ C. chopped bell pepper

- ¼ tsp. onion powder

- ¼ tsp. garlic powder

- 8 ounces of raw lean ground beef

Directions:

1. In a skillet, add seasonings, beef, onion, and bell pepper. Stir and crumble beef till fully cooked and vegetables are soft.

2. Take the skillet off the heat and add cream cheese, mustard, and cheddar cheese, stirring till melted.

3. Pour beef mixture into a bowl and fold in pickles.

4. Roll out egg wrappers and place 1/6th of beef mixture into each one. Moisten egg roll wrapper edges with water. Fold sides to the middle and seal with water.

5. Repeat with all other egg rolls.

6. Place rolls into the air fryer, one batch at a time.

7. Pour into the Oven rack/basket. Place the Rack on the middle-shelf of the Air Fryer Oven. Set temperature to 392°F, and set time to 7 minutes.

Nutrition:

Calories 153 Cal

Fat 4 g

Carbs 0 g

Protein 12 g

Chapter 2. Poultry

13. Lemon Chicken Breasts

Basic Recipe

Preparation Time: 10 minutes

Cooking Time: 30 minutes

Servings: 4

Ingredients:

- 1/4 cup olive oil

- 3 tablespoons garlic, minced

- 1/3 cup dry white wine

- 1 tablespoon lemon zest, grated

- 2 tablespoons lemon juice

- 1 1/2 teaspoons dried oregano, crushed

- 1 teaspoon thyme leaves, minced

- Salt and black pepper

- 4 skin-on boneless chicken breasts

- 1 lemon, sliced

Directions:

1. Whisk everything in a baking pan to coat the chicken breasts well.

2. Place the lemon slices on top of the chicken breasts.

3. Spread the mustard mixture over the toasted bread slices.

4. Press the "Power Button" of Air Fry Oven and turn the dial to select the "Bake" mode.

5. Press the Time button and again turn the dial to set the cooking time to 30 minutes.

6. Now push the Temp button and rotate the dial to set the temperature at 370 degrees F.

7. Once preheated, place the baking pan inside and close its lid.

8. Serve warm.

Nutrition:

Calories 388

Fat 8 g

Carbs 8 g

Protein 13 g

14. Almond Flour Battered Chicken Cordon Bleu

Basic Recipe

Preparation Time: 5 minutes

Cooking Time: 30 minutes

Servings: 2

Ingredients:

- ¼ cup almond flour

- 1 slice cheddar cheese

- 1 slice of ham

- 1 small egg, beaten

- 1 teaspoon parsley

- 2 chicken breasts, butterflied

- Salt and pepper to taste

Directions:

1. Season the chicken with parsley, salt and pepper to taste.

2. Place the cheese and ham in the middle of the chicken and roll. Secure with a toothpick.

3. Soak the rolled-up chicken in egg and dredge in almond flour.

4. Place in the air fryer.

5. Cook for 30 minutes at 350F.

Nutrition:

Calories 1142

Carbs 5.5g

Protein 79.4g

Fat 89.1g

15. Almond Flour Coco-Milk Battered Chicken

Basic Recipe

Preparation Time: 5 minutes

Cooking Time: 30 minutes

Servings: 4

Ingredients:

- ¼ cup coconut milk

- ½ cup almond flour

- 1 ½ tablespoons old bay Cajun seasoning

- 1 egg, beaten

- 4 small chicken thighs

- Salt and pepper to taste

Directions:

1. Preheat the air fryer for 5 minutes.

2. Mix the egg and coconut milk in a bowl.

3. Soak the chicken thighs in the beaten egg mixture.

4. In a mixing bowl, combine the almond flour, Cajun seasoning, salt and pepper.

5. Dredge the chicken thighs in the almond flour mixture.

6. Place in the air fryer basket.

7. Cook for 30 minutes at 350F.

Nutrition:

Calories 590

Carbs3.2g

Protein 32.5 g

Fat 38.6g

16. Basil-Garlic Breaded Chicken Bake

Intermediate Recipe

Preparation Time: 5 minutes

Cooking Time: 30 minutes

Servings: 2

Ingredients:

- 2 boneless skinless chicken breast halves (4 ounces each)

- 1 tablespoon butter, melted

- 1 large tomato, seeded and chopped

- 2 garlic cloves, minced

- 1 1/2 tablespoons minced fresh basil

- 1/2 tablespoon olive oil

- 1/2 teaspoon salt

- 1/4 cup all-purpose flour

- 1/4 cup egg substitute

- 1/4 cup grated Parmesan cheese

- 1/4 cup dry bread crumbs

- 1/4 teaspoon pepper

Directions:

1. In a shallow bowl, whisk well egg substitute and place flour in a separate bowl. Dip chicken in flour, then egg, and then flour. In a small bowl, whisk well the butter, bread crumbs and cheese. Sprinkle over chicken.

2. Lightly grease the baking pan of the air fryer with cooking spray. Place breaded chicken on the bottom of the pan. Cover with foil.

3. For 20 minutes, cook it at 390 F.

4. Meanwhile, in a bowl, whisk well the remaining ingredients.

5. Remove foil from the pan and then pour over the chicken the remaining Ingredients. Cook for 8 minutes. Serve and enjoy.

Nutrition:

Calories 311

Carbs 22.0g

Protein 31.0g

Fat 11.0g

17. BBQ Chicken Recipe from Greece

Basic Recipe

Preparation Time: 5 minutes

Cooking Time: 24minutes

Servings: 2

Ingredients:

- 1 (8 ounces) container fat-free plain yogurt

- 2 tablespoons fresh lemon juice

- 2 teaspoons dried oregano

- 1-pound skinless, boneless chicken breast halves - cut into 1-inch pieces

- 1 large red onion, cut into wedges

- 1/2 teaspoon lemon zest

- 1/2 teaspoon salt

- 1 large green bell pepper, cut into 1 1/2-inch pieces

- 1/3 cup crumbled feta cheese with basil and sun-dried tomatoes

- 1/4 teaspoon ground black pepper

- 1/4 teaspoon crushed dried rosemary

Directions:

1. In a shallow dish, mix well rosemary, pepper, salt, oregano, lemon juice, lemon zest, feta cheese, and yogurt. Add chicken and toss well to coat. Marinate in the ref for 3 hours.

2. Thread bell pepper, onion, and chicken pieces in skewers. Place on skewer rack.

3. For 12 minutes, cook it on 360F. Turnover skewers halfway through cooking time. If needed, cook in batches.

4. Serve and enjoy.

Nutrition:

Calories 242

Carbs 12.3g

Protein 31.0g

Fat 7.5g

18. BBQ Pineapple 'n Teriyaki Glazed Chicken

Basic Recipe

Preparation Time: 5 minutes

Cooking Time: 20 minutes

Servings: 2

Ingredients:

- ¼ cup pineapple juice

- ¼ teaspoon pepper

- ½ cup brown sugar

- ½ cup soy sauce

- ½ teaspoon salt

- 1 green bell pepper, cut into 1-inch cubes

- 1 red bell pepper, cut into 1-inch cubes

- 1 red onion, cut into 1-inch cubes

- 1 Tablespoon cornstarch

- 1 Tablespoon water

- 1 yellow red bell pepper, cut into 1-inch cubes

- 2 boneless skinless chicken breasts cut into 1-inch cubes

- 2 cups fresh pineapple cut into 1-inch cubes

- 2 garlic cloves, minced

- Green onions for garnish

Directions:

1. In a saucepan, bring to a boil salt, pepper, garlic, pineapple juice, soy sauce, and brown sugar. In a small bowl, whisk well, cornstarch and water. Slowly stir into mixture in the pan while whisking constantly. Simmer until thickened, around 3 minutes. Save ¼ cup of the sauce for basting and set aside.

2. In a shallow dish, mix well chicken and the remaining thickened sauce. Toss well to coat. Marinate in the ref for a half hour.

3. Thread bell pepper, onion, pineapple, and chicken pieces in skewers. Place on skewer rack in the air fryer.

4. For 10 minutes, cook on 360F. Turnover skewers halfway through cooking time. And baste with sauce. If needed, cook in batches.

5. Serve and enjoy with a sprinkle of green onions.

Nutrition:

Calories 391 Carbs 58.7g

Protein 31.2g Fat 3.4g

19. BBQ Turkey Meatballs with Cranberry Sauce

Basic Recipe

Preparation Time: 5 minutes

Cooking Time: 20 minutes

Servings: 4

Ingredients:

- 1 ½ tablespoons of water

- 2 teaspoons cider vinegar

- 1 tsp. salt and more to taste

- 1-pound ground turkey

- 1 1/2 tablespoons barbecue sauce

- 1/3 cup cranberry sauce

- 1/4-pound ground bacon

Directions:

1. In a bowl, mix well with hands the turkey, ground bacon and a tsp. of salt. Evenly form into 16 equal-sized balls.

2. In a small saucepan, boil cranberry sauce, barbecue sauce, water, cider vinegar, and a dash or two of salt. Mix well and simmer for 3 minutes.

3. Thread meatballs in skewers and baste with cranberry sauce. Place on skewer rack in the air fryer.

4. For 15 minutes, cook it on 360F. Every after 5 minutes of cooking time, turnover skewers and baste with sauce. If needed, cook in batches.

5. Serve and enjoy.

Nutrition:

Calories 217

Carbs 11.5g

Protein 28.0g

Fat 10.9g

20. Buffalo Style Chicken Dip

Basic Recipe

Preparation Time: 5 minutes

Cooking Time: 10 minutes

Servings: 4

Ingredients:

- 1 (8 ounce) package cream cheese, softened

- 1 tablespoon shredded pepper Jack cheese

- 1/2 pinch cayenne pepper for garnish

- 1/2 pinch cayenne pepper, or to taste

- 1/4 cup and 2 tablespoons hot pepper sauce (such as Frank's Reshoot®)

- 1/4 cup blue cheese dressing

- 1/4 cup crumbled blue cheese

- 1/4 cup shredded pepper Jack cheese

- 1/4 teaspoon seafood seasoning (such as Old Bay®)

- 1-1/2 cups diced cooked rotisserie chicken

Directions:

1. Lightly grease the baking pan of the air fryer with cooking spray. Mix in cayenne pepper, seafood seasoning, crumbled blue cheese, blue cheese dressing, pepper Jack, hot pepper sauce, cream cheese, and chicken.

2. For 15 minutes, cook it at 390 F.

3. Let it stand for 5 minutes and garnish with cayenne pepper.

4. Serve and enjoy.

Nutrition:

Calories 405

Carbs 3.2g

Protein 17.1g

Fat 35.9g

Chapter 3. Seafood

21. Grilled Sardines

Preparation Time: 5 minutes

Cooking Time: 20 minutes

Servings: 4

Ingredients:

- 5 sardines

- Herbs of Provence

Directions:

1. Preheat the air fryer to 160C.

2. Spray the basket and place your sardines in the basket of your fryer.

3. Set the timer for 14 minutes. After 7 minutes, remember to turn the sardines so that they are roasted on both sides.

Nutrition:

Calories: 189g Fat: 10g

Carbs: 0g Sugars: 0g

Protein: 22g

Cholesterol: 128mg

22. Buttered Salmon

Basic Recipe

Preparation Time: 5 minutes

Cooking Time: 10 minutes

Servings: 2

Ingredients:

- 2 salmon fillets (6-oz)

- Salt and ground black pepper, as required

- 1 tbsp. butter, melted

Directions:

1. Season each salmon fillet with salt and black pepper and then coat with the butter. Arrange the salmon fillets onto the greased cooking tray.

2. Arrange the drip pan in the bottom of the Instant Vortex Air Fryer Oven cooking chamber. Select "Air Fry" and then adjust the temperature to 360 °F. Set the time for 10 minutes and press "Start".

3. When the display shows "Add Food" insert the cooking tray in the center position. When the display shows "Turn Food" turn the salmon fillets.

4. When cooking time is complete, remove the tray from the Vortex Oven. Serve hot.

Nutrition:

Calories: 276

Carbs: 0g

Fat: 16.3g

Protein: 33.1g

23. Lemony Salmon

Basic Recipe

Preparation Time: 5 minutes

Cooking Time: 10 minutes

Servings: 2

Ingredients:

- 1 tbsp. of fresh lemon juice

- ½ tbsp. olive oil

- Salt and ground black pepper, as required

- 1 garlic clove, minced

- ½ tsp. fresh thyme leaves, chopped

- 2 (7-oz) Salmon fillets

Directions:

1. In a bowl, add all ingredients, except for the salmon, and mix well. Add the salmon fillets and coat with the mixture generously.

2. Arrange the salmon fillets onto a lightly greased cooking rack, skin-side down. Arrange the drip pan in the bottom of the Instant Vortex Air Fryer Oven cooking chamber. Select "Air

Fry" and then adjust the temperature to 400 °F. Set the time for 10 minutes and press "Start".

3. When the display shows "Add Food" insert the cooking rack in the bottom position. When the display shows "Turn Food" turn the fillets.

4. When the cooking time is complete, remove the tray from the Vortex Oven. Serve hot.

Nutrition:

Calories: 297

Carbs: 0.8g

Fat: 15.8g

Protein: 38.7g

24. Miso Glazed Salmon

Basic Recipe

Preparation Time: 5 minutes

Cooking Time: 10 minutes

Servings: 4

Ingredients:

- 1/3 cup sake

- ¼ cup sugar

- ¼ cup red miso

- 1 tbsp. low-sodium soy sauce

- 2 tbsp. vegetable oil

- 4 (5-oz) Skinless salmon fillets, (1-inch thick)

Directions:

1. Place the sake, sugar, miso, soy sauce, and oil into a bowl and beat until thoroughly combined. Rub the salmon fillets with the mixture generously. In a plastic Ziploc bag, place the salmon fillets with any remaining miso mixture.

2. Seal the bag and refrigerate to marinate for about 30 minutes. Grease a baking dish that will fit in the Vortex Air Fryer Oven. Remove the salmon fillets from the bag and shake off the

excess marinade. Arrange the salmon fillets into the prepared baking dish.

3. Arrange the drip pan in the bottom of the Instant Vortex Air Fryer Oven cooking chamber. Select "Broil" and Set the time for 5 minutes.

4. When the display shows "Add Food" insert the baking dish in the center position.

5. When the display shows "Turn Food" do not turn the food. When cooking time is complete, remove the baking dish from the Vortex Oven. Serve hot.

Nutrition:

Calories: 335

Carbs: 18.3g

Fat: 16.6g

Protein: 29.8g

25. Spiced Tilapia

Basic Recipe

Preparation Time: 5 minutes

Cooking Time: 12 minutes

Servings: 2

Ingredients:

- ½ Tsp. lemon pepper seasoning

- ½ tsp. Garlic powder

- ½ tsp onion powder

- Salt and ground black pepper, as required

- 2 (6-oz) tilapia fillets

- 1 tbsp. olive oil

Directions:

1. In a small bowl, mix together the spices, salt, and black pepper. Coat the tilapia fillets with oil and then rub with spice mixture. Arrange the tilapia fillets onto a lightly greased cooking rack, skin-side down.

2. Arrange the drip pan in the bottom of the Instant Vortex Air Fryer Oven cooking chamber. Select "Air Fry" and then adjust

the temperature to 360 °F. Set the time for 12 minutes and press "Start".

3. When the display shows "Add Food" insert the cooking rack in the bottom position. When the display shows "Turn Food" turn the fillets.

4. When cooking time is complete, remove the tray from the Vortex Oven. Serve hot.

Nutrition:

Calories: 206

Carbs: 0.2g

Fat: 8.6g

Protein: 31.9g

26. Crispy Tilapia

Basic Recipe

Preparation Time: 5 minutes

Cooking Time: 15 minutes

Servings: 2

Ingredients:

- ¾ cup cornflakes, crushed

- 1 (1-oz.) packet, dry ranch-style dressing mix

- 2½ tbsp. vegetable oil

- 2eggs

- 4 (6-oz) tilapia fillets

Directions:

1. In a shallow bowl, beat the eggs. In another bowl, add the cornflakes, ranch dressing, and oil and mix until a crumbly mixture forms. Dip the fish fillets into the egg and then coat with the cornflake mixture.

2. Arrange the tilapia fillets onto the greased cooking tray. Arrange the drip pan in the bottom of the Instant Vortex Air Fryer Oven cooking chamber. Select "Air Fry" and then adjust

the temperature to 355 °F. Set the time for 14 minutes and press "Start".

3. When the display shows "Add Food" insert the cooking tray in the center position. When the display shows "Turn Food" turn the tilapia fillets. When cooking time is complete, remove the tray from the Vortex Oven. Serve hot.

Nutrition:

Calories: 291

Carbs: 4.9g

Fat: 14.6g

Protein: 34.8g

27. Spicy Catfish

Basic Recipe

Preparation Time: 5 minutes

Cooking Time: 15 minutes

Servings: 4

Ingredients:

- 2 tbsp cornmeal polenta

- 2 tsp cajun seasoning

- ½ tsp paprika

- ½ tsp garlic powder

- Salt, as required

- 2 (6-oz) catfish fillets

- 1 tbsp. olive oil

Directions:

1. In a bowl, mix together the cornmeal, Cajun seasoning, paprika, garlic powder, and salt. Add the catfish fillets and coat evenly with the mixture. Now, coat each fillet with oil.

2. Arrange the fish fillets onto a greased cooking rack and spray with cooking spray. Arrange the drip pan in the bottom of the

Instant Vortex Air Fryer Oven cooking chamber. Select "Air Fry" and then adjust the temperature to 400 °F. Set the timer for 14 minutes and press "Start".

3. When the display shows "Add Food" insert the cooking rack in the center position. When the display shows "Turn Food" turn the fillets.

4. When cooking time is complete, remove the rack from the Vortex Oven. Serve hot.

Nutrition:

Calories: 32

Carbs: 6.7g

Fat: 20.3g

Protein: 27.3g

28. Tuna Burgers

Basic Recipe

Preparation Time: 5 minutes

Cooking Time: 6 minutes

Servings: 4

Ingredients:

- 7 Oz canned tuna

- 1 large egg

- ¼ cup breadcrumbs

- 1 tbsp. Mustard

- ¼ tsp garlic powder

- ¼ tsp onion powder

- ¼ tsp. cayenne pepper

- Salt and ground black pepper, as required

Directions:

1. Add all the ingredients into a bowl and mix until well combined. Make 4 equal-sized patties from the mixture.

2. Arrange the patties onto a greased cooking rack. Arrange the drip pan in the bottom of the Instant Vortex Air Fryer Oven cooking chamber. Select "Air Fry" and then adjust the temperature to 400 °F. Set the time for 6 minutes and press "Start".

3. When the display shows "Add Food" insert the cooking rack in the center position.

4. When the display shows "Turn Food" turn the burgers.

5. When the cooking time is complete, remove the tray from the Vortex Oven. Serve hot.

Nutrition:

Calories: 151

Carbs: 6.3g

Fat: 6.4g

Protein: 16.4g

29. Crispy Prawns

Basic Recipe

Preparation Time: 5 minutes

Cooking Time: 10 minutes

Servings: 4

Ingredients:

- 1egg

- ½ lb. crushed nacho chips

- 12prawns, peeled and deveined

Directions:

1. In a shallow dish, beat the egg. In another shallow dish, place the crushed nacho chips. Coat the prawn into the egg and then roll into nacho chips.

2. Arrange the coated prawns onto 2 cooking trays in a single layer. Arrange the drip pan in the bottom of the Instant Vortex Air Fryer Oven cooking chamber. Select "Air Fry" and then adjust the temperature to 355 °F. Set the time for 8 minutes and press "Start".

3. When the display shows "Add Food" insert 1 tray in the top position and another in the bottom position. When the display shows "Turn Food" do not turn the food but switch the

position of cooking trays. When cooking time is complete, remove the trays from the Vortex Oven. Serve hot.

Nutrition:

Calories: 386

Carbs: 36.1g

Fat: 17g

Protein: 21g

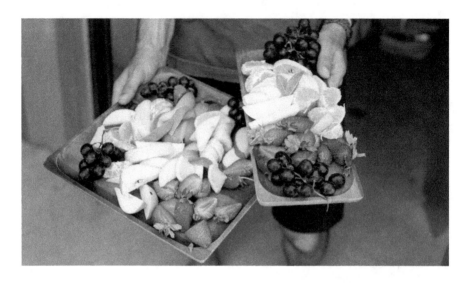

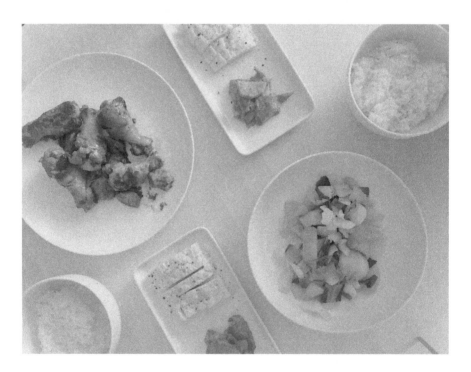

Chapter 4. Vegetables and Sides

30. Broccoli-Rice 'n Cheese Casserole

Basic Recipe

Preparation Time: 5 minutes

Cooking Time: 30 minutes

Servings: 4

Ingredients:

- 1 (10 ounces) can chunk chicken, Dry out

- 1 cup uncooked instant rice

- 1 cup water

- 1/2 (10.75 ounces) can condensed cream of chicken soup

- 1/2 (10.75 ounces) can condensed cream of mushroom soup

- 1/2 cup milk

- 1/2 small white onion, chopped

- 1/2-pound processed cheese food

- 2 tablespoons butter

- 8-ounce frozen chopped broccoli

Directions:

1. Lightly grease the baking pan of the air fryer with cooking spray. Add water and bring to a boil at 390°F. Stir in rice and cook for 3 minutes.

2. Stir in processed cheese, onion, broccoli, milk, butter, chicken soup, mushroom soup, and chicken. Mix well. Cook for 15 minutes at 390F, fluff mixture and continue cooking for another 10 minutes until tops are browned. Serve and enjoy.

Nutrition:

Calories 752

Carbs 82.7g

Protein 36.0g

Fat 30.8g

31. Baked Rice, Black Bean and Cheese

Intermediate Recipe

Preparation Time: 5 minutes

Cooking Time: 1 hour

Servings: 4

Ingredients:

- 1 cooked skinless boneless chicken breast halves, chopped

- 1 cup shredded Swiss cheese

- 1/2 (15 ounces) can black beans, Dry out

- 1/2 (4 ounces) can diced green chili peppers, Dry out

- 1/2 cup vegetable broth

- 1/2 medium zucchini, thinly sliced

- 1/4 cup sliced mushrooms

- 1/4 teaspoon cumin

- 1-1/2 teaspoons olive oil

- 2 tablespoons and 2 teaspoons diced onion

- 3 tablespoons brown rice

- 3 tablespoons shredded carrots

- Ground cayenne pepper to taste

- Salt to taste

Directions:

1. Lightly grease the baking pan of the air fryer with cooking spray. Add rice and broth. Cover pan with foil cook for 10 minutes at 390°F. Lower heat to 300°F and fluff rice. Cook for another 10 minutes. Let it stand for 10 minutes and transfer it to a bowl and set it aside.

2. Add oil to the same baking pan. Stir in onion and cook for 5 minutes at 330°F.

3. Stir in mushrooms, chicken, and zucchini. Mix well and cook for 5 minutes

4. Stir in cayenne pepper, salt, and cumin. Mix well and cook for another 2 minutes

5. Stir in ½ of the Swiss cheese, carrots, chilies, beans, and rice. Toss well to mix. Evenly spread in pan. Top with remaining cheese.

6. Cover pan with foil. Cook for 15 minutes at 390°F and then remove foil and cook for another 5 to 10 minutes or until tops are lightly browned. Serve and enjoy.

Nutrition: Calories 337Carbs 11.5gProtein 25.3g

Fat 21.0g

32. Beefy 'n Cheesy Spanish Rice Casserole

Intermediate Recipe

Preparation Time: 10 minutes

Cooking Time: 50 minutes

Servings: 3

Ingredients:

- 2 tablespoons chopped green bell pepper

- 1 tablespoon chopped fresh cilantro

- 1/2-pound lean ground beef

- 1/2 cup water

- 1/2 teaspoon salt

- 1/2 teaspoon brown sugar

- 1/2 pinch ground black pepper

- 1/3 cup uncooked long grain rice

- 1/4 cup finely chopped onion

- 1/4 cup chili sauce

- 1/4 teaspoon ground cumin

- 1/4 teaspoon Worcestershire sauce

- 1/4 cup shredded Cheddar cheese

- 1/2 (14.5 ounces) can canned tomatoes

Directions:

1. Lightly grease the baking pan of the air fryer with cooking spray. Add ground beef.

2. For 10 minutes, cook on 360°F. Halfway through cooking time, stir and crumble beef. Discard excess fat,

3. Stir in pepper, Worcestershire sauce, cumin, brown sugar, salt, chili sauce, rice, water, tomatoes, green bell pepper, and onion. Mix well. Cover pan with foil and cook for 25 minutes. Stirring occasionally

4. Give it one last good stir, press down firmly, and sprinkle cheese on top.

5. Cook uncovered for 15 minutes at 390°F until tops are lightly browned.

6. Serve and enjoy with chopped cilantro.

Nutrition:

Calories 346 Cal

Fat 19.1 g

Carbs 0 g

Protein 18.5 g

33. Easy Air Fried Roasted Asparagus

Basic Recipe

Preparation Time: 5 minutes

Cooking Time: 10 minutes

Servings: 4

Ingredients:

- 1 bunch fresh asparagus

- 1 ½ tsp. herbs de Provence

- Fresh lemon wedge (optional)

- 1 tablespoon olive oil or cooking spray

- Salt and pepper to taste

Directions:

1. Wash asparagus and trim off hard ends. Drizzle with asparagus with olive oil and add seasonings

2. Place asparagus in the air fryer and cook on 360F for 6 to 10 minutesDrizzle with squeezed lemon over roasted asparagus.

Nutrition: Calories 46 Protein 2g Fat 3g Carbs 1g

34. Air Fryer Roasted Broccoli

Basic Recipe

Preparation Time: 5 minutes

Cooking Time: 10 minutes

Servings: 4

Ingredients:

- 1 tsp. herbs de Provence seasoning (optional)

- 4 cups fresh broccoli

- 1 tablespoon olive oil

- Salt and pepper to taste

Directions:

1. Drizzle with or spray broccoli with olive and sprinkle seasoning throughout

2. Spray air fryer basket with cooking oil, place broccoli, and cook for 5-8 minutes on 360F

3. Open air fryer and examine broccoli after 5 minutes because different fryer brands cook at different rates.

Nutrition: Calories 61 Fat 4g Protein 3g Carbs 4g

35. Air Fryer Veggie Quesadillas

Basic Recipe

Preparation Time: 20 minutes

Cooking Time: 20 minutes

Servings: 4

Ingredients:

- 4 sprouted whole-grain flour tortillas (6-in.)

- 1 cup sliced red bell pepper

- 4 ounces reduced-fat Cheddar cheese, shredded

- 1 cup sliced zucchini

- 1 cup canned black beans, Dry out, and rinsed (no salt)

- Cooking spray

- 2 ounces plain 2% reduced-fat Greek yogurt

- 1 teaspoon lime zest

- 1 Tbsp. fresh juice (from 1 lime)

- ¼ tsp. ground cumin

- 2 tablespoons chopped fresh cilantro

- 1/2 cup Dry out refrigerated pico de gallo

Directions:

1. Place tortillas on the work surface, sprinkle 2 tablespoons shredded cheese over half of each tortilla, and top with cheese on each tortilla with 1/4 cup each red pepper slices, zucchini slices, and black beans. Sprinkle evenly with remaining 1/2 cup cheese.

2. Fold tortillas over to form half-moon shaped quesadillas, lightly coat with cooking spray, and secure with toothpicks.

3. Lightly spray air fryer basket with cooking spray. Place 2 quesadillas in the basket, and cook at 400°F for 10 minutes until tortillas are golden brown and slightly crispy, cheese is melted, and vegetables are slightly softened. Turn quesadillas over halfway through cooking.

4. Repeat with remaining quesadillas. Meanwhile, stir yogurt, lime juice, lime zest, and cumin in a small bowl. Cut each quesadilla into wedges and sprinkle with cilantro.

5. Serve with 1 tablespoon cumin cream and 2 tablespoons pico de gallo each.

Nutrition:

Calories 291

Fat 8g

Protein 17g

Carbs 36g

Chapter 5. Meat

36. Medium-Rare Beef Steak

Basic Recipe

Preparation Time: 5 minutes

Cooking Time: 6 minutes

Servings: 4

Ingredients:

- 1-3cm thick beef steak

- 1 tablespoon olive oil

- Salt and pepper to taste

Directions:

1. Preheat your air fryer to 350°Fahrenheit.

2. Coat the steak with olive oil on both sides and season both sides with salt and pepper.

3. Place the steak into the baking tray of the air fryer and cook for 3-minutes per side.

Nutrition:

Calories 445 Fat 21g,

Carbs 0g, Protein 59.6g

37. Garlic Pork Chops

Basic Recipe

Preparation Time: 5 minutes **Cooking Time:** 16 minutes

Servings: 4

Ingredients:

- 4 pork chops

- 1 tablespoon coconut butter

- 2 teaspoons minced garlic cloves

- 1 tablespoon coconut butter

- 2 teaspoons parsley, chopped

- Salt and pepper to taste

Directions:

1. Preheat your air fryer to 350°Fahrenheit.

2. In a bowl, mix the coconut oil, seasonings, and butter. Coat the pork chops with this mixture. Place the chops on the grill pan of your air fryer and cook them for 8-minutes per side.

Nutrition: Calories 356 Fat 30g Carbs 2.3g Protein 19g

38. Mustard Pork Balls

Basic Recipe

Preparation Time: 5 minutes

Cooking Time: 15 minutes

Servings: 4

Ingredients:

- 7-ounces of minced pork

- 1 teaspoon of organic honey

- 1 teaspoon Dijon mustard

- 1 tablespoon cheddar cheese, grated

- 1/3 cup onion, diced

- Salt and pepper to taste

- A handful of fresh basil, chopped

- 1 teaspoon garlic puree

Directions:

1. In a bowl, mix the meat with all of the seasonings and form balls.

2. Place the pork balls into the air fryer and cook for 15-minutes at 392°Fahrenheit.

Nutrition:

Calories 121

Fat 6.8g

Carbs 2.7g

Protein 11.3g

39. Crispy Mustard Pork Tenderloin

Preparation Time: 10 minutes

Cooking Time: 12-16 minutes

Servings: 4

Ingredients:

- 3 tablespoons low-sodium grainy mustard

- 2 teaspoons olive oil

- ¼ teaspoon dry mustard powder

- 1 (1-pound) pork tenderloin, silverskin, and excess fat trimmed and discarded

- 2 slices low-sodium whole-wheat bread, crumbled

- ¼ cup ground walnuts

- 2 tablespoons cornstarch

Directions:

1. In a small bowl, stir together the mustard, olive oil, and mustard powder. Spread this mixture over the pork.

2. On a plate, mix the bread crumbs, walnuts, and cornstarch. Dip the mustard-coated pork into the crumb -mixture to coat.

3. Air-fry the pork for 12 to 16 minutes, or until it registers at least 145°F on a meat thermometer. Slice to serve.

Nutrition:

Calories: 239

Fat: 9g

Saturated Fat: 2g

Protein: 26g

Carbohydrates: 15g

Sodium: 118m

Fiber: 2g

Sugar: 3g

40. Apple Pork Tenderloin

Preparation Time: 10 minutes

Cooking Time: 14-19 minutes

Servings: 4

Ingredients:

- 1 (1-pound) pork tenderloin, cut into 4 pieces

- 1 tablespoon apple butter

- 2 teaspoons olive oil

- 2 Granny Smith apples or Jonagold apples, sliced

- 3 celery stalks, sliced

- 1 onion, sliced

- ½ teaspoon dried marjoram

- ⅓ cup apple juice

Directions:

1. Rub each piece of pork with apple butter and olive oil.

2. In a medium metal bowl, mix the pork, apples, celery, onion, marjoram, and apple juice.

3. Place the bowl into the air fryer and roast for 14 to 19 minutes, or until the pork reaches at least 145°F on a meat thermometer and the apples and vegetables are tender. Stir once during cooking. Serve immediately.

Nutrition:

Calories: 213

Fat: 5g

Saturated Fat: 1g

Protein: 24g

Carbohydrates: 20g

Sodium: 88mg

Fiber: 3g

Sugar: 15g

Chapter 6. Soup and Stews

41. Bacon and Cauliflower Soup

Basic Recipe

Preparation Time: 10 minutes

Cooking Time: 20 minutes

Servings: 4

Ingredients:

- 2 tablespoons of butter

- 4 cups of chicken stock

- 1 large onion, chopped

- 4 potatoes, chopped

- 3 cups of cauliflower florets

- ½ cup of heavy cream

- 1 tablespoon of salt

- 1 tablespoon of black pepper

- 12 slices of bacon, crisp fried

Directions:

1. Set the Instant Vortex on the air fryer to 375 degrees F for 5 minutes, put the bacon, potatoes, and cauliflower in the cooking tray. Insert the cooking tray in the Vortex when it displays "Add Food". Remove from the Vortex when cooking time is complete. Put the butter in a wok and add the onions.

2. Sauté it for about 3 minutes and then stir in the bacon mixture and the chicken stock. Secure the lid of the wok and cook for about 10 minutes on medium heat. Pour this mixture into an immersion blender and puree it. Ladle out in a bowl to serve.

Nutrition:

Calories 344

Protein 8.3g

Carbs 44.1g

Fat 16.7g

42. Basil Tomato Soup

Basic Recipe

Preparation Time: 5 minutes

Cooking Time: 15 minutes

Servings: 4

Ingredients:

- 1 onion, roughly sliced

- 1 potato, roughly diced

- ½ cup of tomatoes

- 2 tablespoons of tomato paste

- 2 tablespoons of sun-dried tomatoes

- 1 tablespoon of basil leaves, freshly chopped

- 1 carrot, roughly chopped

- 4 cups of water

- Salt and black pepper to taste

- 2 tablespoons of butter

Directions:

1. Set the Instant Vortex on the air fryer to 375 degrees F for 5 minutes. Put the tomatoes, potato, carrot, and sun-dried tomatoes in the cooking tray. Insert the cooking tray in the Vortex when it displays "Add Food". Remove from the Vortex when cooking time is complete. Put the butter in a wok and add the tomato mixture and onions.

2. Sauté it for about 3 minutes and then stir in the remaining ingredients. Secure the lid of the wok and cook for about 12 minutes on medium heat. Puree the contents of the soup with an immersion blender and serve hot.

Nutrition:

Calories 239

Protein 4.2g

Carbs 29.6g

Fat 12.8g

43. Pumpkin Tomato Soup

Basic Recipe

Preparation Time: 10 minutes

Cooking Time: 20 minutes

Servings: 4

Ingredients

- 4 tablespoons of pumpkin puree

- 1 cup of tomatoes, chopped

- 4 cups of water

- 1 onion, roughly sliced

- 3 tablespoons of tomato paste

- 1 teaspoon of pumpkin spice powder

- 4 tablespoons of butter

- 1 carrot, roughly chopped

- 1 potato, roughly diced

- 3 tablespoons of sun-dried tomatoes

- 2 pinches of black pepper

- 2 teaspoons of salt

Directions:

1. Set the Instant Vortex on the air fryer to 375 degrees F for 5 minutes. Put the tomatoes, carrots, potato, and sun-dried tomatoes in the cooking tray.

2. Insert the cooking tray in the Vortex when it displays "Add Food".

3. Remove from the Vortex when cooking time is complete. Put the butter in a wok and add the onions.

4. Sauté for about 3 minutes and then stir in the tomato mixture along with the remaining ingredients.

5. Secure the lid of the wok and cook for about 12 minutes on medium heat.

6. Pour this mixture into an immersion blender and puree it. Ladle out in a bowl to serve.

Nutrition:

Calories 190

Protein 2.8g

Carbs 18.5g

Fat 12.7g

Chapter 7. Snack, Appetizer, Side

44. Date & Walnut Bread

Intermediate Recipe

Preparation Time: 15 minutes

Cooking Time: 35 minutes

Servings: 5

Ingredients:

- 1 cup dates, pitted and sliced

- ¾ cup walnuts, chopped

- 1 tablespoon instant coffee powder

- 1 tablespoon hot water

- 1¼ cups plain flour

- ¼ teaspoon salt

- ½ teaspoon baking powder

- ½ teaspoon baking soda

- ½ cup condensed milk

- ½ cup butter, softened

- ½ teaspoon vanilla essence

Directions:

1. In a large bowl, add the dates, butter, and top with the hot water.

2. Set aside for about 30 minutes.

3. Dry out well and set aside.

4. In a small bowl, add the coffee powder and hot water and mix well.

5. In a large bowl, mix together the flour, baking powder, baking soda, and salt.

6. In another large bowl, add the condensed milk and butter and beat until smooth.

7. Add the flour mixture, coffee mixture, and vanilla essence and mix until well combined.

8. Fold in dates and ½ cup of walnut.

9. Line a baking pan with lightly greased parchment paper.

10. Place the mixture into the prepared pan and sprinkle with the remaining walnuts.

11. Press the "Power Button" of the Air Fry Oven and turn the dial to select the "Air Crisp" mode.

12. Press the Time button and again turn the dial to set the cooking time to 35 minutes.

13. Now push the Temp button and rotate the dial to set the temperature at 320 degrees F.

14. Press the "Start/Pause" button to start.

15. When the unit beeps to show that it is preheated, open the lid.

16. Arrange the pan in "Air Fry Basket" and insert it in the oven.

17. Place the pan onto a wire rack to cool for about 10 minutes.

18. Carefully invert the bread onto a wire rack to cool completely before slicing.

19. Cut the bread into desired-sized slices and serve.

Nutrition:

Calories 593

Fat 32.6 g

Carbs 69.4 g

Protein 11.2 g

45. Brown Sugar Banana Bread

Intermediate Recipe

Preparation Time: 15 minutes

Cooking Time: 30 minutes

Servings: 4

Ingredients:

- 1 egg

- 1 ripe banana, peeled and mashed

- ¼ cup milk

- 2 tablespoons canola oil

- 2 tablespoons brown sugar

- ¾ cup plain flour

- ½ teaspoon baking soda

Directions:

1. Line a very small baking pan with a greased parchment paper.

2. In a small bowl, add the egg and banana and beat well.

3. Add the milk, oil, and sugar and beat until well combined.

4. Add the flour and baking soda and mix until just combined.

5. Place the mixture into the prepared pan.

6. Press the "Power Button" of the Air Fry Oven and turn the dial to select the "Air Crisp" mode.

7. Press the Time button and again turn the dial to set the cooking time to 30 minutes.

8. Now push the Temp button and rotate the dial to set the temperature at 320 degrees F.

9. Press the "Start/Pause" button to start.

10. When the unit beeps to show that it is preheated, open the lid.

11. Arrange the pan in "Air Fry Basket" and insert it in the oven.

12. Place the pan onto a wire rack to cool for about 10 minutes.

13. Carefully invert the bread onto a wire rack to cool completely before slicing.

14. Cut the bread into desired-sized slices and serve.

Nutrition:

Calories 214

Fat 8.7 g

Carbs 29.9 g

Protein 4.6 g

46. Cinnamon Banana Bread

Basic Recipe

Preparation Time: 15 minutes

Cooking Time: 20 minutes

Servings: 8

Ingredients:

- 1 1/3 cups flour

- 2/3 cup sugar

- 1 teaspoon baking soda

- 1 teaspoon baking powder

- 1 teaspoon ground cinnamon

- 1 teaspoon salt

- ½ cup milk

- ½ cup olive oil

- 3 bananas, peeled and sliced

Directions:

1. In the bowl of a stand mixer, add all the ingredients and mix well.

2. Grease a loaf pan.

3. Place the mixture into the prepared pan.

4. Press the "Power Button" of the Air Fry Oven and turn the dial to select the "Air Crisp" mode.

5. Press the Time button and again turn the dial to set the cooking time to 20 minutes.

6. Now push the Temp button and rotate the dial to set the temperature at 330 degrees F.

7. Press the "Start/Pause" button to start.

8. When the unit beeps to show that it is preheated, open the lid.

9. Arrange the pan in "Air Fry Basket" and insert it in the oven.

10. Place the pan onto a wire rack to cool for about 10 minutes.

11. Carefully invert the bread onto a wire rack to cool completely before slicing.

12. Cut the bread into desired-sized slices and serve.

Nutrition:

Calories 295

Fat 13.3g

Carbs 44 g Protein 3.1 g

47. Banana & Walnut Bread

Basic Recipe

Preparation Time: 15 minutes

Cooking Time: 25 minutes

Servings: 10

Ingredients:

- 1½ cups self-rising flour

- ¼ teaspoon bicarbonate of soda

- 5 tablespoons plus 1 teaspoon butter

- 2/3 cup plus ½ tablespoon caster sugar

- 2 medium eggs

- 3½ oz. walnuts, chopped

- 2 cups bananas, peeled and mashed

Directions:

1. In a bowl, mix together the flour and bicarbonate of soda.

2. In another bowl, add the butter and sugar and beat until pale and fluffy.

3. Add the eggs, one at a time, along with a little flour, and mix well.

4. Stir in the remaining flour and walnuts.

5. Add the bananas and mix until well combined.

6. Grease a loaf pan.

7. Place the mixture into the prepared pan.

8. Press the "Power Button" of the Air Fry Oven and turn the dial to select the "Air Crisp" mode.

9. Press the Time button and again turn the dial to set the cooking time to 10 minutes.

10. Now push the Temp button and rotate the dial to set the temperature at 355 degrees F.

11. Press the "Start/Pause" button to start.

12. When the unit beeps to show that it is preheated, open the lid.

13. Arrange the pan in "Air Fry Basket" and insert it in the oven.

14. After 10 minutes of cooking, set the temperature at 338 degrees F for 15 minutes.

15. Place the pan onto a wire rack to cool for about 10 minutes.

16. Carefully invert the bread onto a wire rack to cool completely before slicing.

17. Cut the bread into desired-sized slices and serve.

Nutrition:

Calories 270

Fat 12.8 g

Carbs 35.5 g

Protein 5.8 g

48. Banana & Raisin Bread

Intermediate Recipe

Preparation Time: 15 minutes

Cooking Time: 40 minutes

Servings: 6

Ingredients:

- 1½ cups cake flour

- 1 teaspoon baking soda

- ½ teaspoon ground cinnamon

- Salt to taste

- ½ cup vegetable oil

- 2 eggs

- ½ cup sugar

- ½ teaspoon vanilla extract

- 3 medium bananas, peeled and mashed

- ½ cup raisins, chopped finely

Directions:

1. In a large bowl, mix together the flour, baking soda, cinnamon, and salt.

2. In another bowl, beat well eggs and oil.

3. Add the sugar, vanilla extract, and bananas and beat until well combined.

4. Add the flour mixture and stir until just combined.

5. Place the mixture into a lightly greased baking pan and sprinkle with raisins.

6. With a piece of foil, cover the pan loosely.

7. Press the "Power Button" of the Air Fry Oven and turn the dial to select the "Air Bake" mode.

8. Press the Time button and again turn the dial to set the cooking time to 30 minutes.

9. Now push the Temp button and rotate the dial to set the temperature at 300 degrees F.

10. Press the "Start/Pause" button to start.

11. When the unit beeps to show that it is preheated, open the lid.

12. Arrange the pan in "Air Fry Basket" and insert it in the oven.

13. After 30 minutes of cooking, set the temperature to 285 degrees F for 10 minutes.

14. Place the pan onto a wire rack to cool for about 10 minutes.

15. Carefully invert the bread onto a wire rack to cool completely before slicing.

16. Cut the bread into desired-sized slices and serve.

Nutrition:

Calories 448

Fat 20.2 g

Carbs 63.9 g

Protein 6.1 g

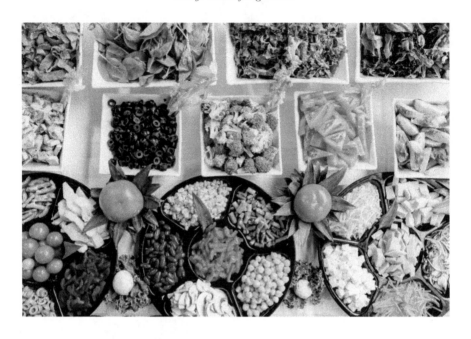

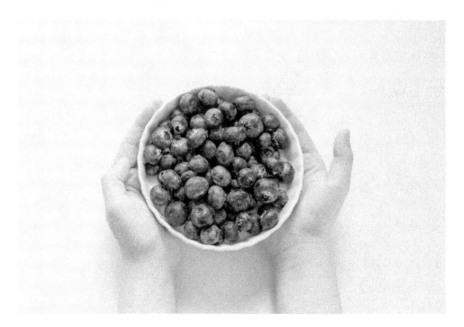

Chapter 8. Desserts

49. Apple Dumplings

Preparation Time: 10 minutes

Cooking Time: 25 minutes

Servings: 4

Ingredients:

- 2 tbsp. melted coconut oil

- 2 puff pastry sheets

- 1 tbsp. brown sugar

- 2 tbsp. raisins

- 2 small apples of choice

Directions:

1. Ensure your air fryer oven is preheated to 356 degrees.

2. Core and peel apples and mix with raisins and sugar. Place a bit of apple mixture into puff pastry sheets and brush sides with melted coconut oil. Place into the air fryer. Cook 25 minutes, turning halfway through. It will be golden when done.

Nutrition: Calories – 367Protein – 2 g.Fat – 7 g.Carbs – 10 g.

50. Chocolate Donuts

Preparation Time: 5 minutes

Cooking Time: 20 minutes

Servings: 8-10

Ingredients:

- (8-ounce) can jumbo biscuits

- Cooking oil

- Chocolate sauce, such as Hershey's

Directions:

1. Separate the biscuit dough into 8 biscuits and place them on a flat work surface. Use a small circle cookie cutter or a biscuit cutter to cut a hole in the center of each biscuit. You can also cut the holes using a knife.

2. Grease the basket with cooking oil.

3. Place 4 donuts in the air fryer oven. Do not stack. Spray with cooking oil. Cook for 4 minutes.

4. Open the air fryer and flip the donuts. Cook for an additional 4 minutes.

5. Remove the cooked donuts from the air fryer oven, then repeat for the remaining 4 donuts.

6. Drizzle chocolate sauce over the donuts and enjoy while warm.

Nutrition:

Calories – 181

Protein – 3 g.

Fat – 98 g.

Carbs – 42 g.

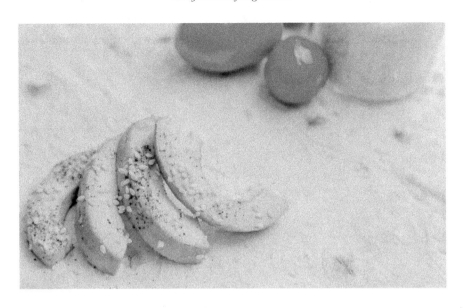

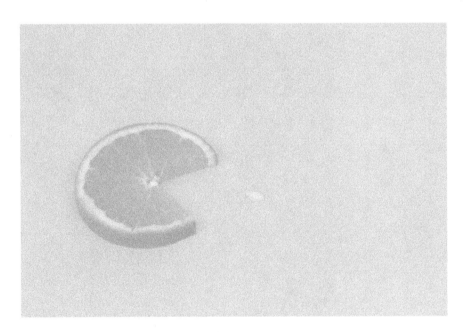

Conclusion

Now that you reached the end of this book, those recipes will give you different vibes and make you feel like an expert chef by using your Instant Vortex Air Fryer. Try the recipes in this book and give yourself and your family something to look forward to even on weekdays.

Air Fry: using this program to cook oil-free, crispy food, whether it's coated meat or fries, everything can be fried in its Air fryer basket.

Toast: the temp/time dial used to set the temperature and cooking time can be used to select the bread slices and their brownness when they need to be toasted using the Toast cooking program of the Instant Air Fryer toaster oven.

Bake: it is used to bake cakes, brownies, or bread in a quick time.

Broil: the broiler's settings provide direct top-down heat to crisp meat, melt cheese, and caramelizes the vegetables and fruits. It has the default highest temperature, which is 450 degrees F.

Roast: this cooking program is suitable for roasting meats and vegetables.

Slow Cooker: the Slow Cook program lets you adjust greater cooking time and lowest temperatures based on the requirements.

Reheat: using this mode, the users can warm up leftover food without overcooking the food.

Dehydrate: low-temperature heat is regulated to effectively remove moisture from foods, thus giving perfect crispy veggie chips, jerky, and dehydrated fruits.

For a longer usage or its span, always remember that the Instant Air Fryer Toaster Oven must be cleaned after every cooking session like any other cooking appliance. It is important to keep the inside of the oven germs free all the time. The food particles that are stuck at the base or on the oven's walls should be cleaned after every session using the following steps:

Unplug the Instant Air Fryer toaster oven and allow it to cool down completely. Keep the door open while it cools down. Remove all the trays, dripping pan, steel racks, and other accessories from inside the oven.

Place the removable parts of the oven in the dishwasher and wash them thoroughly. Once these accessories are washed, all of them dry out completely. Meanwhile, take a clean and slightly damp cloth to clean the inside of the oven.

Wipe all the internal walls of the oven using this cloth. Be gentle while you do the wiping. Use another cloth to clean the exterior of the appliance. Wipe off all the surfaces. Now that everything is clean, you can place the steel racks and dripping pan back to their position for the next cooking session.

CPSIA information can be obtained
at www.ICGtesting.com
Printed in the USA
BVHW042213130421
604819BV00009BA/978

9 781914 350733